Pass or Fail Dating

Date. Eliminate. Ameliorate.

A dating upgrade guide, by T. Goodwyn.

ISBN: 978-0-9847246-7-3

Copyright © 2024 by T. Goodwyn, all rights reserved.

First Edition

Table of Contents

Introduction	1
The Honeymoon Dates	5
Honeymoon-is-Over Dating	15
Seasoned Daters	29
A Kiss Under the Porch Light	35
Relationship Rules Reference	39
A Note from the Author	43

Pass or Fail Dating

A definitive guide to an upgraded way of dating and finding that compatible partner. The Pass or Fail Dating method works for any dating adult, regardless of gender, age, race, culture, orientation, personality, or any fun mix of these.

T. Goodwyn: Respected psychotic analyst and experienced relationship ameliorator.

Pass or Fail Dating

Introduction

Unless you're a fresh face to the dating scene, there's a good chance you've experienced some disappointments. Maybe you've been seeing a potential life partner for a while, but are now beginning to question the reasons you've been overlooking some annoying behavior. Or maybe you've noticed how other people seem to enjoy dating while you are not. Instead of having fun, is your patience being tested?

For many, that's exactly what dating someone is: a test. An exam with inadequate study guides and a complex set of rules and variables that require the navigational skills of Ferdinand Magellan.

Some daters are happy-go-lucky. They are in it for the fun of it and don't care if they do or do not get along with someone. If they had fun, they'll go on another date with them. If not, they move on. These are the ones who are probably dating multiple people simultaneously, which might work for a while, but will eventually cause conflicts.

If you're spending time with potential life partners because you want to get to know them well, you may think you have time for complicated grading systems and/or lists of pros and cons, but this approach involves a lot of wasted time. Your time is precious. Consider streamlining the experience. The Pass or Fail method is simple and easy to adopt.

Near the end of a date, or shortly thereafter, take a moment and try to imagine spending the rest of your life with that potential partner. If you think you could possibly make a life with them, or you're not sure yet, they passed that test. Plan the next date.

If you can't imagine spending the rest of your life with that potential partner, move on. This is the foundation of Pass or Fail Dating. Move on. Eliminate. It's okay. You don't have to spend time dating someone who isn't right for you. You don't have to be with someone you don't really like because disappointing them or breaking up with them seems more difficult than staying together.

Moving on will avoid getting yourself into a situation where you are secretly hoping a potential partner will change some unacceptable behavior. *They are probably not going to change.* If you don't move on, days of indecision might become weeks, or even months.

Pass or Fail Dating

And, unless you're a mental health professional, it's not your responsibility to change people. Waiting on potential partners to make improvements will probably be a complete waste of your time, which you could be spending looking for someone compatible. What if that perfect companion came into your life while you were waiting for someone incompatible to improve their bad behavior?

Lingering with the wrong potential partner is not only a waste of your precious time, it also makes future dating more difficult. The longer you stay together with incompatible partners, the harder future dating becomes for you, for them, *and* for all *their* future potential partners. Ending a relationship as soon as you realize it's not viable is crucial, so you'll want to know about their bad habits and poor behaviors early in the dating process.

Claiming that people don't change seems harsh, but that's reality. Instead of changing, most "iffy" people simply find a potential partner who is desperate enough to tolerate bad behavior. If someone *does* change, it's because so many people have broken up with them that they finally understand their behavior is a problem. So, move on. Do your part.

Try to give the iffy people feedback. They need to know what drives others away so that they stand a chance of improving their disorders enough to find someone decent. Sadly, if they don't make improvements, they will eventually find that incredibly tolerant person who will put up with them, but deserves better.

Keep in mind that it may take several dates, or weeks, or even *months* to realize that you don't want to spend the rest of your life with the person you've been dating. That's okay. It's not too late to move on. Don't waste any more time. Go find someone worthy.

If you familiarize yourself with the simple guidelines in this collection, you will likely learn enough about people to move on before you feel invested in a relationship. If your potential partner only has one bad behavior that irritates you, or just a few minor things you feel you can overlook, you might make the relationship work, but that is what it will be. Work. On *your* part. And drama. Work and drama. Do you want that in your life? Is any potential partner worth all that? *You* must decide.

Pass or Fail Dating

The Honeymoon Dates

People inherently want to impress potential life partners, so for those first few dates, they are typically on their best behavior. This time is often referred to as The Honeymoon Phase. Unfortunately, this portrays many in a more flattering light than they deserve.

You will probably prefer their best behavior, but if you can discover the true nature of your potentials sooner, you might be able to save yourself some time and resources.

So, how do you implement Pass or Fail dating? Let's get started.

- Buy your potential life partner a box of chocolates. Seriously. Make sure it has a good assortment, and then pay attention. Or check back later or the next day. If they smashed or pinched chocolates to reveal whatever is in the center, but then returned some to the container because they didn't want it, that person is too picky or too selfish to be in a relationship.

Okay, that might seem a little harsh for such a minor infraction, but is it? The underlying reasons feeding this behavior is a little disturbing. They want someone else to eat their refuse, or otherwise deal with the mess they made. Should they pass or fail?

If you choose to ignore this behavior, be prepared for more selfishness. That potential life partner better be worth it.

- Few things are as disrespectful as one person blatantly interrupting another. Nothing says, "I don't care about your thoughts or anything you say," like cutting someone off in mid-sentence to interject some random thought. If your date interrupts you more than a couple of times, you might want to excuse yourself, say goodbye, and cut off all contact.

Let's meet our friends Goodwyn and Iffy. (Get it? A good one and another who is a little iffy?)

Iffy: "So! Tell me a little about yourself. Where are you from?"

Goodwyn: "Well, I was born in Springfield, but moved to Fairview when—"

Iffy, after a dramatic gasp: "My first job was in Fairview!" Iffy goes on and on about an uninteresting job so long that they both forget that Goodwyn was in the middle of a sentence.

Goodwyn, patiently waiting for Iffy to stop talking...

- There is a similar behavior that is uncommon, but is still interrupting. It's just *disguised* interrupting. This behavior is usually carried out by habitual attention seekers. If your date begins speaking loudly before or while entering a room where people are talking, that means the attention-seeker doesn't care about anyone else's thoughts.

Iffy, coming into a room where others are engaged in conversations: "Where's my phone?"

Goodwyn looks around.

Iffy: "Has *any*one seen my phone?"

Goodwyn whips out their phone and calls Iffy.

Iffy: "Woo! It was in my pocket!"

Iffy, after dinner, interrupting several casual conversations over dessert: "Where's my phone? Has anyone seen my phone?"

Goodwyn: *Sigh*

If you realize a potential life partner is the type with a self-perceived need to always be the center of attention, excuse yourself, say goodbye, and cut off all contact. If you don't, that person will eventually begin to annoy you. Every day.

- If you have access to their kitchen, look for another telltale sign indicating whether your potential mate is, or is not a planner. Look at their loaf of bread, if they have one. Again, seriously. If the "heel" of the bread is gone, that likely means they ate it first, without caring or, even worse, without understanding that the slice of bread at the end serves to keep the rest of the loaf from drying out. If your potential life partner doesn't understand how to plan for the future with something as simple as a loaf of bread, they better be worth the frustration this shortcoming will cause.

Pass or Fail Dating

- Try to get a look inside your potential life partner's refrigerator, if you can, or their bathroom, to check the lids of containers to see if they have been replaced properly. It is a problem if the lids on the toothpaste, the ketchup bottle, or the fabric softener, or whatever, are not tightened snugly. If those lids are loose, or even worse, just placed on top of the container with no effort made to screw them on, that person probably doesn't care about consequences. Or the future. They may not be capable of planning ahead at all.

If this complaint seems petty to you, be assured, it is not. You are getting a glimpse into the future. *Your* future, if you allow it.

Goodwyn, at a trendy new local restaurant: "Iffy, could you pass me the BBQ sauce?"

Iffy: "Certainly." Iffy passes the bottle of BBQ sauce, but fails to warn Goodwyn that they had only placed the lid on top, and did not screw it down.

Goodwyn: "Thanks." Goodwyn takes the bottle and attempts to give it a good shake, but of course, the lid comes off and BBQ sauce splatters all over the table and a brand-new shirt, purchased specifically for the date they are on.

Iffy laughs, albeit good-naturedly.

Goodwyn does not laugh.

If you choose to ignore this lazy behavior, that potential life partner better be worth it.

- Speaking of toothpaste and the bathroom, while you're there, look for smears of toothpaste on the towel. Notice if, after brushing, they used the towel to wipe the toothpaste from their mouth instead of washing their mouth with water first. If the telltale smears are there, that is a good indication that they don't care about anyone who needs to use the towel after them. The same is probably going to be true for other aspects of their life. They don't care who must deal with the careless spoils they leave in their wake.

    If you choose to ignore this seemingly-harmless behavior, that potential life partner better be worth you often not even being an afterthought.

- If you have free reign of the house, you might as well check their closet, too. You can tell a lot about someone from their closet. The longer they've lived there, the more you'll be able to discover. Look for clothes hangers with nothing on them. If they are scattered throughout the closet, still hanging where clothing was hastily ripped off them, this also means they probably don't plan well for the future. If the empty hangers are all in one spot, you know they took the piece of clothing down, removed it from the hanger, then hung it in the same place with all the other empty hangers. When it's time to do laundry, retrieving the hangers is simple, and not a frustrating hunt between all the clothing in the closet.

Weekly frustration is something you'll have to live with someday, as *you* will become the one gathering all those hangers on wash day. That potential life partner better be worth the resentment you'll harbor.

- If your date's place is a mess, a future home with them will also be a mess. That's something you'll have to live with. That potential life partner better be worth cleaning up after, or hiring weekly housecleaners. For the rest of your life.

- Throughout the dating process, always listen closely for hints that your potential partner is superstitious. The superstitious ones sometimes drive sane people nuts. However, don't confuse the occasional common saying like "knock on wood" with true superstitious beliefs. If they are overly religious, or religious at all when you are not, these disparities will eventually clash and cause problems. But even if you and your potential life partner are the rare ones who see eye-to-eye on religion, other superstitious beliefs will likely be irritating.

    Iffy: "I prayed *hard*, and swore that if I got that promotion at work, I'd be vegan for a year!"

    Goodwyn: "And, that's why you think you got the promotion?"

    Iffy: "Yes! It *has* to be!"

Pass or Fail Dating

Goodwyn: "I think you probably got that promotion because you're the best employee there."

Iffy, horrified: "No! It was because I prayed."

Goodwyn: "So, there are others who do that job better than you?"

Iffy: "Well, no."

Goodwyn: "Others were probably praying for that job, too. Right?"

Iffy: "Of course, but *I've* been doing this job a lot longer than anyone else and have an extensive knowledge base."

Goodwyn, nodding wisely: "Hmm…"

Iffy, missing the point entirely: "And YOU are going to be vegan with me."

Goodwyn, no longer nodding: "Hmmmm…"

- Your potential partner will likely have a combination of their parents' or guardians' worst traits, although it might not be apparent, at first. If possible, meet their parents or whoever raised them early in the dating process. Spend some time with them, and notice their worst behaviors and habits. Some people wind up having the best traits of their parents or guardians. Those are the partners you want. But if you even see a hint of the inherited bad behaviors, it will get worse, not better. Bad habits *rarely* get better. That potential life partner better be worth it.

Pass or Fail Dating

Honeymoon-is-Over Dating

If your potential life partner has passed enough dates for the two of you to make it through the honeymoon phase, you may now be allowing each other to see more of each other's personality traits. This is a good progression! However, be aware that poor behavior patterns may still be revealed. That's okay, too. You want to identify those as early in a relationship as possible.

Maybe you're spending time at each other's place, or possibly even fooling around. Either of these things is fine, of course. You do what's right for you and let others do what's right for them.

Romantic, weekend getaways are a good way to get to know one another. People can get to know one another better when they spend extended times with each other in a car, an airplane, or a hotel room. This is a good way to find out if the person you're dating is truly a potential life partner. Just be ready to recognize imperfect behaviors while paying attention to disclosures and exposures.

- Treating your potential life partner the same way they treat you is a good compatibility test.

If their mimicked behavior irritates them or they get upset, you should probably think about abandoning that relationship as soon as possible. If you stay with them after knowing that their behavior even irritates them, that potential partner better be worth the inequitable treatment.

- If your date takes a towel and/or the toilet paper from the hotel room when you check out, or tries to "cheat" housekeeping out of extra lotion, shampoo and conditioner, that greed is something you'll have to live with every time you go on vacation. That potential life partner better be worth it.

- I'll be the first to admit that toilet paper should have little to do with determining whether a relationship is viable or not, but if your potential partner puts the toilet paper roll on backwards, eventually, this will irritate you every time you go to the bathroom. What do you do? Do you turn it around so that it's on the roll correctly? Do you leave it and stifle your irritation? Do you talk to them about something that is seemingly so trivial, but leads to animosities and resentments?

These are the things that might go through your head, *every, time,* you use the bathroom. Do not underestimate the proper placement of the loose end. It's something you'll have to live with. That potential life partner better be worth the multiple-times-per-day irritation.

- The household thermostat is another good way to measure compatibility. Your potential life partner needs to have a basic understanding of how a thermostat works. If they don't already know, there is little likelihood that explaining it will help them understand that the air coming out of the vents does not get colder when you adjust the temperature to a lower setting.

  It's true.

  Whether the air conditioner is set to fifty degrees or seventy degrees, the air coming out of the vents will be the same temperature. The difference is, the A/C turns off when the thermometer in the thermostat reaches the designated temperature. And yes, the heater is the same way, only in reverse. The wilder they are with the setting, the less likely they are to understand the common thermostat. This is something you'll have to live with. That potential life partner better be worth it.

Iffy: "I am SO hot!" Gets up, adjusts the thermostat to 62°.

Iffy, a half an hour later: "I am SO cold!" Gets up, adjusts thermostat to 80°.

Goodwyn: "Can we just set the thermostat to the temperature that you want?"

Iffy: "I *still* don't understand what you're talking about. Why does it have to be so complicated?"

Goodwyn: *Sigh. Is this potential life partner worth the irritation and higher utility bills?*

- Potential life partners who shake a leg or are forever jittery will drive you nuts. Imagine being on the couch, or maybe in bed, and your potential is absentmindedly shaking a leg. You probably won't be able to get comfortable. Or get to sleep until they fall asleep.

Iffy: Shaking a leg while binge-watching the latest season of that streaming murder-show series they wanted to watch.

Iffy: Still shaking that leg two episodes later.

Goodwyn: "Is there an earthquake happening?"

Iffy: With both legs shaking now, "No, it's just me. I *have* to move."

Goodwyn: "You're shaking the whole couch."

Iffy: Leg movements increase noticeably.

That potential life partner better be worth a lifetime of discomfort and/or irritation.

- If your potential partner watches those "reality" shows that feature a group of people who argue and fight like grade school children in every show, chances are, that's how your life will be. They better be worth it.

- For TV watchers, the remote control is often a source of contention. If your potential life partner insists that they be the one in control of it, or if they never put the remote back in the same place, forcing you to search for it every time you want to watch a show, you better get used to it. Buying another remote won't help. Both will end up in their possession, and that's how it will be for the rest of your life. They better be worth it.

- Cooking meals together can be revealing, too. Pay attention to how your potential life partner throws spices in the pot or bowl. See if they dump it all into one pile, or spread the spices around in the pot or skillet so it is not clumped up. If they dump it all into one pile, and then stir it in, the spices will never get mixed in to all the ingredients. Some bites will be over-seasoned and some will be bland. If your potential partner can't plan well enough to properly season a dish, their ability to plan may be compromised altogether. They better be worth the failures to plan.

- Car keys and mobile phones present a similar problem. If your potential life partner constantly misplaces their phone, or can't remember where they last put their keys every time they want to leave the house, their entire life is probably disorganized, as well.

Unfortunately, few people can be retrained to always put their keys back on a hook by the door, or a staging area on the way to the door. That potential life partner better be worth it.

- Back seat drivers will make you crazy, too. I'm not talking about the people who yell "Look out!" when a car pulls out in front of you, or you're about to back into something in a parking lot. They *are* the people who state the obvious about traffic conditions, even when it would be impossible for the driver to not see it. And of course, back seat drivers are more likely to be in the front seat, than the back.

    Iffy: "There's a crosswalk right up here, be careful, sometimes people cross the street there."

    Iffy: "Brake lights!"

    Iffy: "You're following a little too closely."

    Iffy: "Okay, the light turned red, slow down now."

    Goodwyn: *Sigh.*

That potential life partner better be worth the irritation you'll experience every time you travel together.

- A lot of people like to remove their shoes when they come in from outside. If your potential life partner often "forgets" and walks across your carpet with their dirty shoes, that could be more of a lack of respect than a matter of absentmindedness. However, if they take off their shoes, but leave them right in the middle of the doorway for others to trip over, that stretches beyond a lack of respect. This probably means that they are completely oblivious to the needs of others. That potential life partner's oblivion better be worth it.

- If your potential life partner watches you sit down, then asks you to do something that involves you getting back up, that's fine. But if they do that often, it's a form of manipulation. If your potential life partner is worth you being manipulated, get used to it.

- Pay attention to dirty dishes. Of course, help wash them, or help rinse and load them into the dishwasher. But pay attention to how your potential life partner loads the dishwasher. If they load the dishwasher without rinsing the dishes first, or without rinsing them thoroughly, you're either dealing with general laziness, or a lack of understanding of what a dishwasher does.

If dishes retrieved from a dishwasher are stained or discolored by food, that means organic particles have been absorbed into the surface of the dish. Those food particles will spoil as quickly as food left out on the counter. The stains do not remain "sterile" because they were once run through the dishwasher. This concept is another one of those things where people probably cannot be retrained. They better be worth eating from perpetually dirty dishes.

- A subset of the issues with dishes is the goal of loading the dishwasher. The reason dishes go in the dishwasher is to get them clean. The goal is *not* to see how many dishes can be stacked into one load. The *only* goal is to get the dishes clean. If your potential partner overloads the dishwasher, they either do not understand the simple mechanics of a dishwasher, or they care more about completing the job than getting the dishes clean. Finishing chores may *always* be more important to them than the quality of the completed task. That potential life partner better be worth it.

- Continuing with the theme of the kitchen, if your potential life partner does not know the difference between a cup towel and a hand towel, it is likely too late. You can rarely teach adults the difference.

  Most organized kitchens sport two different sets of towels. One for dishes and another for hands and other kitchen uses. Not all kitchens have two sets though, so you need to remember that once you dry your hands off on a kitchen towel, it becomes a hand towel and is not to be used on clean dishes. A cup towel is what you use to dry dishes that have been washed or removed from the dishwasher. You don't want the towel you used to dry your hands all over your clean dishes. If your potential life partner is oblivious to all this, they better be worth the disgust and irritation.

Pass or Fail Dating

- When you're hanging out on a weekend, and your potential life partner makes coffee in one of the older style coffee makers where you put the grounds in the filter and the water drips through to a pot, pay attention. If they put too much coffee in the filter so that the first pot is way too strong, simply so that they can make a second pot with the used grounds, this is a problem.

  "Second coffee" is not frugal, it's just the wrong way to do it. The first pot will have zero chance of being delicious (unless you're from France or Italy, of course) and the second pot will be too weak. Making coffee this way makes people feel clever so, sadly, it's unlikely that the second coffee people will ever learn to use the correct amount of coffee grounds. That potential life partner better be worth a lifetime of bad coffee, or worth keeping an environmentally unfriendly, single-use coffee maker in the kitchen.

- Iffy: Adds cream, sugar, and a splash of hazelnut syrup to their coffee, stirs it, and then places the spoon face up on Goodwyn's clean counter so that doctored-up coffee settles into the bottom of the spoon. Iffy then slurps their hot coffee loudly.

Goodwyn: Cringes, picks up the spoon, and places it onto a napkin, upside down, so that the coffee, sugar and dairy do not dry in the bottom of the spoon.

Iffy: May or may not notice, and might either think, *Geez, what a control freak*, or, hopefully, *Oh! What a good idea!*

If your potential life partner doesn't put the spoon down upside down after stirring their goodies into their cup, the coffee or tea settles in the bottom of the spoon. It often dries quickly, too, because the spoon is warm from the hot beverage. It's a little bit gross, especially if your potential partner has different tastes than you. If someone else wants to use that spoon to stir their coffee or tea again, they will have to rinse that mess out first.

This seemingly-insignificant behavior is likely an insight into how well they plan or consider the future. When you point out this simplicity and they begin placing the spoon upside down, there's a chance they might learn to plan for the future. If they continue to place that spoon so that their beverage settles into the bottom, there is little chance that planning is a skill in which they excel.

Keep in mind that if you make these kinds of suggestions more than once or twice, you *will* sound like a control freak. You don't want to be with someone you feel you have to control before you can be happy, and you *sure* don't want someone to think you're a control freak. Your potential life partner needs to be both willing to learn and able to teach.

- To get a better idea of compatibility, you might want to see how well you relax together. When the nights turn cool, take your potential life partner to the hot springs or a romantic spot with a jacuzzi. Make it a weekend trip, if you can. Just sit back in the relaxing water and see if they relax with you. If they do not, but pester you instead, you better get used to that irritation.

Goodwyn, relaxing in a hot spring pool: "Aaahh. Perfect. Thanks for coming up here with me."

Iffy, already irritated with the idea of sitting still: "Perfect? We walked through snow to get here."

Goodwyn: "Well, we *are* in the mountains. Just look at that sunset."

Iffy: "I am *not* a fan of snow."

Goodwyn: "Good thing we're in this cozy warm water, then, huh? Come on, let's snuggle."

Iffy: "Are there grizzly bears around here?"

Goodwyn: "Nope. Try to relax with me?"

Iffy: "Is that an ear hair? Let me get that for you."

Goodwyn: *Sigh.*

If the hot springs are something you enjoy, your potential life partner better be worth giving up these kinds of pleasures.

Seasoned Daters

If your potential life partner has passed enough of the honeymoon-is-over dates, you might be spending a lot of time together. Perhaps you've already introduced them to friends and family, or maybe you're even participating in the occasional sleepover. If any of that is true, especially if there is any cohabitation involved, it's time to get into more serious relationship issues.

- Rarely can two or more people agree on everything. I'm sure there are people who have read this book up to this point who have disagreed with some of the points listed. In relationships, disagreements sometimes lead to arguments. Moreso for some than others. How you handle arguments in your relationship is paramount. If your potential life partner must always have the last word in an argument, that is a problem. If you can't even get in the last word by saying "I'm sorry," or "you're right," then that is a *serious* problem. That potential life partner better be worth you never getting your way.

- If you are the one who always apologizes after a disagreement or argument, that might be a problem, too. Yes, it could mean that you are the one causing the arguments, but it could also mean that your potential life partner is unwilling to compromise or admit they are wrong. If you are always the one to apologize after an argument, chances are, they might very well always consider you to be wrong. Try not to apologize after an argument to see if your potential partner will make the initiative to make amends. If they do not, there is a good chance they *never* will, even when you both know they are wrong. That potential life partner better be worth a life of no compromises.

- A potential life partner who uses profanities in the presence of children are probably going to be a problem. If they shout profanities at other drivers, or at the TV, they may have some anger issues, which will also be problematic. That's something you'll either have to live with or successfully maneuver into therapy. That potential life partner better be worth it.

Pass or Fail Dating

- If a potential takes on a couple of unpleasant household tasks, or maybe a few, but does little else to help maintain the home, beware. They may be taking on the distasteful responsibilities so that they will have less work to do overall. There is also a good chance that they are doing them so that they can refer to those good deeds later, when it is most convenient for them. They may feel like they can get away with being responsible for far less than you, or possibly get away with being mean or manipulative, simply by reminding you that *they* are doing the most difficult or unpleasant chores.

  If you mention how unfair or unequal the distribution of daily tasks is, they may make a huge production about how difficult their portion is, so that you will be reluctant to approach the subject again. If they do not respond well to a suggestion of taking on more chores, that person may not be the best partner for you. Or anyone. You must decide if that potential life partner is worth it.

- Even though every couple argues occasionally, if your potential life partner purposefully misinterprets things you say, or puts a spin on your words that you obviously didn't intend, apparently just for the sake of arguing, get used to it, or move on. Be aware that a lot of people would rather *win* than *resolve*. This antisocial behavior rarely improves. That potential life partner better be worth it.

- When your potential life partner needs help with things, help them! And don't be afraid to ask for help sometimes, too. However, if they look over your shoulder while you're performing a task that you do *not* need help with, they are probably trying to "supervise" your work. With this type of person, you will always take a subservient role in that relationship. So, you guessed it, you better be sure you are okay with that potential life partner thinking they are your boss.

- So, you've been spending the night together? Good for you, but, after the fun, what happens? If they roll over and drag all the covers with them, it might just mean that they are not used to being in bed with someone, which is not a bad thing. *Or*, it might mean that they have no regard for anyone else's comfort. You'll have to decide which it is. As with all the issues listed here, a discussion (or dozen) might improve the situation, although that's not likely. If the problem persists, you'll have to decide if that potential life partner is worth the nightly irritation of having the covers yanked off your body.

- Far too often, video games are relationship killers. If someone would rather spend their time online trying to level up, or defeat some virtual "friend" than spend time with you, then so be it. Either learn to live with that and maybe join them, or find your own preferably-productive pastime, or simply move on. If you choose to remain in that relationship, that potential life partner better be worth the isolation you will feel.

- Some potential life partners have alcohol or substance abuse problems. If you discover this about them, there are only two choices. Years, or perhaps decades of lost jobs, extreme frustration, and all your money going down the drain or up in smoke, and to legal expenses, *or* just move on. That sounds harsh but dealing with expensive DUIs (or worse) is infinitely harsher.

Trust logic. You want a partner who chooses to channel their disposable money into viable investments and memorable vacations.

- Worth mentioning are the obvious things most dating self-help manuscripts cover: Money, cheating, bad sex, trust, communication, and, more recently in dating evolution, iPhone users vs. Android users. These are all things that can cause irreconcilable differences. (Okay, your choice of mobile phone probably won't cause severe issues, but it can be irritating.) Choose your potential life partner carefully. If they don't pass a date, don't schedule another. Eliminate and ameliorate.

A Kiss Under the Porch Light

A lot of readers probably realized this earlier, but for those who have not, let me tell you now. All the scenarios discussed in this book are just as often about you, my precious reader, as they are about potential partners. Chances are, *you* do some, or maybe even most of the things listed. It's true, and that's okay. No one's perfect. Just know that you *can* change and evolve, and you will need to if you want to be the best life partner you can be.

Everyone has irritating personality traits. I do, you do, your friends and family do, and so will everyone you date. If either or both of you bring enough positive aspects to the relationship, a lot of these issues can be forgiven, or ignored.

Please understand though, that only a *little* bad behavior tends to overshadow a disproportionate number of good traits. It takes significantly more good qualities to balance the scale of compatibility. Also, if you are guilty of more than three or four of the issues described in this book, you may only have two choices. You can either modify those behaviors, or lower your own standards. If you perpetuate bad behaviors even after you've become aware of them, you will probably have to settle on some mediocre potential partner who is willing to tolerate your flaws.

If you are one of the rare givers, and not one of the more common takers, good for you! But how do you know if your potential life partner is a giver or a taker? You might want to test that out before your next date. And are they even capable of making changes? Can they evolve? Choose a topic that might be a deal breaker, or just something about them that irritates you, and try to get them to change. Pick an issue listed in this book, or something that's more personal to you, and discuss it with your potential partner.

For example, explain to them that flushing the toilet with the lid open sprays a microscopic mist of whatever is in the toilet all over the bathroom and, to a lesser extent, the entire home. (Disgusting, right?) If they still leave the lid up when they flush, or worse, if they openly reject your request as nonsense, they may be incapable of change. Too stubborn to be in a relationship with you. Don't be surprised if they are not able to evolve. Remember, most people cannot, or will not, change their bad behaviors.

While pursuing or maintaining a relationship, remember that *you* are far more likely to change undesirable behaviors than is a potential life partner. Finding someone who does not need to change is the key.

Date. Eliminate. Ameliorate.

T. Goodwyn

Relationship Rules Reference

- Financial problems are the most common cause of stress and resentments in relationships. Get ahead of that. Early in co-habitation situations, create a budget. Build in a buffer for unexpected expenses and, this part is essential, include saving at least 25% of your income for retirement. Enter that budget in a spreadsheet, review it quarterly, adjust as required, and stick to it. (Yes, 25%.)

- Alcohol and recreational drug use are the second most common causes of relationship problems. Avoid both completely, no matter how much money it saves you.

- It takes *two* to argue. It's better to simply not argue. Ever. Say what's on your mind, clarify anything unclear, and move on, even if you have not convinced your partner that your point is correct. You might realize later that you *did* convince them, but losing an argument makes them feel weak. Or, you might realize *you* were wrong. It happens, so just don't argue. Ever.

- It takes *one* to end an argument, and it will probably be up to you to end arguments, so learn to do that well. This includes the daunting task of not causing or having residual negative feelings.

- At appropriate times, ask yourself what's more important; being right, or being loving and supportive?

- Your significant other cannot be expected to control their emotional outbursts, which means it's out of your control, too. Know that most people, some more than others, are overly dramatic. Do not participate in the tantrums or drama. Getting drawn in will only prolong the discomfort.

- When your potential life partner is in the middle of an emotional outburst, do not take any of the negative things they say too seriously. There may be some truth to their rants, but they are likely exaggerating how they feel at that moment. Try to hear what they are attempting to say. Somewhere in that outburst is a coded message, and *you* will need to remain in control of your emotions so you can decipher it.

- Your significant other might try to punish you for whatever mistakes you have made. It's what angry people do. If you want the relationship to work, you may need to let them believe they have successfully punished you.

- Let your potential life partner express their negative emotions. Deal with them when *they* want to discuss them. If they don't get the chance to deal with negative emotions consciously, on their own terms, they will shed those negative emotions unconsciously, and you won't enjoy that.

- When they need to vent, listen. No matter how hard it is or how wrong they are, just listen. Even if they raise their voice or even screech. Eventually, they might realize how wrong they are. Sometimes they will even admit it. When they do, don't gloat. If you gloat, they will never admit to being wrong again.

- No matter how much you give, or how hard you try, your efforts will probably not be fully reciprocated. Overall, you'll be happier if you accept this fact. In every relationship (that works) there are either two givers or a giver and a taker. Unfortunately, most people are selfish. There are a lot more takers than givers. Two takers sometimes try to settle into relationships which usually produces stressful situations. All this means that if you want a relationship to work you *may* have to take the initiative to be more of a giver.

- Remember that patience expends energy. If you are constantly consuming more energy to maintain your relationship than your potential life partner, you might be better off finding someone who requires less maintenance. Date, eliminate, and ameliorate.

- If you feel like the person you are dating is a potential life partner, but they could use some improvement, you might want to ask them to read this book. An early beta-reader listened to the audio version on a road trip with their spouse, and they said it "helped them *both* immensely."

A Note from the Author

If you learned *any*thing from Pass or Fail Dating, please take couple of minutes out of your busy day to log on to wherever you purchased this book and give it a rating. (Hint: Being generous with the stars is the most meaningful way to tell authors you enjoyed or appreciated their hard work.) And if you have a *few* minutes to spare, please leave a review, too. I'd love your honest feedback. *Your* words can make a difference in future books.

Thank you!

T

T. Goodwyn

Pass or Fail Dating
Date, eliminate, ameliorate.

Copyright © 2024 by T. Goodwyn, all rights reserved.

www.ingramcontent.com/pod-product-compliance
Lightning Source LLC
Chambersburg PA
CBHW062105290426
44110CB00022B/2723